The Simple and Tasty

Fruit & Veggie

Smoothie Diet

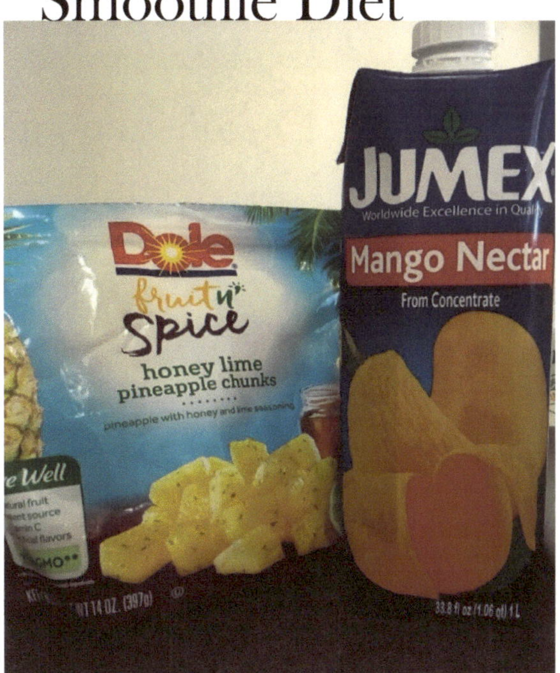

Take the 30-Day Challenge to Weightloss

Energy Boosting * Cleansing* Weight loss Formulas

By: Heaven Salter

Table of Contents

Mangos, peaches, strawberries, bananas all of these yummy fruits are not only healthy sugar items but are a great source of healing and for balancing a diet. There have been many types of diets out there that require complicated food monitoring or aren't compatible with our daily lives. By far the easiest and most affordable diet plan has to be the fruit and veggie diet. Not only does it taste great but eating daily fruits and vegetables balance you out and they are essential in staying truly healthy. In fact, certain fruits and vegetables can even fight off and put off diseases and help alleviate stress.

Have you ever heard the phrase," An apple a day, keeps the doctor away,"? It really is as simple as eating regular fruits and vegetables daily in order to stay healthy and fight off sicknesses. A little exercise here and there doesn't hurt either. In fact, once you start this smoothie diet you will gain so much energy that you won't have to drag yourself to the gym. You will find yourself doing pushups on your living room floor or jumping jacks just because. I know this may sound silly, but when you feel good, you start to think clearly. Your whole way of being will change. You will feel happier, more upbeat and you will start to live a little more.

I've laid out this book in simple terms. You will get simple recipes with simple ingredients that take really little effort and will be within any budget you set. All the smoothies will take less then 5 minutes to prepare and just minutes to blend and enjoy. In order to be most effective with this diet, I recommend you replace 1 meal a day with a smoothie for the first week. Then you will step it up to 2 smoothies a day for the next 5 days. After a week's time you will notice that this will start becoming a routine and you will begin to enjoy it.

It really doesn't matter which smoothie combinations you tackle. The important thing is that you follow the recipe and replace your meals. My suggestion for your first trial at this is to replace breakfast with a smoothie. If you are not a breakfast person, then start drinking a smoothie for breakfast. Then for lunch eat something substantial but healthy. Next for dinner pull back and eat something light like soup or a light meal. The purpose of this diet is not to stress you out about your eating habits. It is only meant to retrain your eating habits and things take time. Pace yourself no one can replace 3 meals a day with smoothies cold turkey. That is why I define this plan in a simple and non-aggressive way. Therefore, start with one smoothie replacement. Next week jump to 2 smoothie replacements and by the third week when you jump to 3 smoothie drinks as your meals you won't even think twice about it.

While you are going about the meal replacement process anytime you get hungry or need to snack on something eat some fruit or blend another smoothie. The idea is that you fill your stomach with more liquid than solid and if you make your smoothies properly they will start to curb your appetite.

Now by the 4th week you are to go back to a normal diet except you will replace only 1 meal with a smoothie and just before bed you will drink a green smoothie or a detox smoothie.

You will continue this new eating method until you have achieved your goal or have changed your lifestyle by choice. Remember to enjoy the process along the way. Now let's dive into the fruits and veggies smoothie diet benefits. All foods have healing properties and the right combination of them can save lives-the natural way!

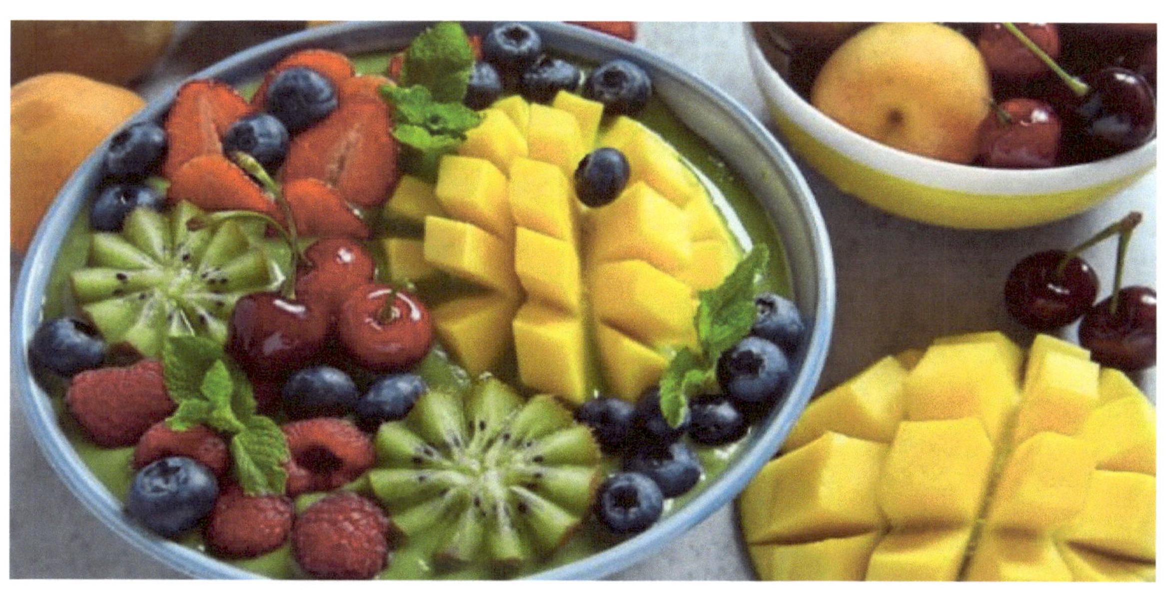

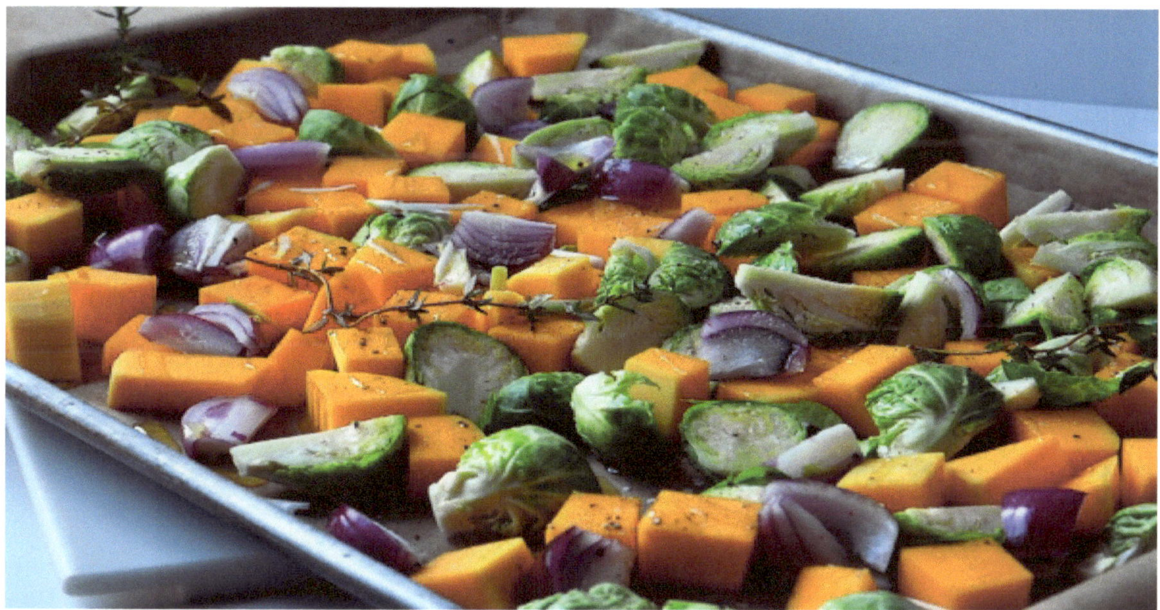

The most potent medicine is eating the skins off your fruit. Most of us instinctively begin to peel our fruits and throw away the most important part. Apple skins, cherry skins and lemon skins have all proven to not only boost the immune system but fight off cancers and other diseases.

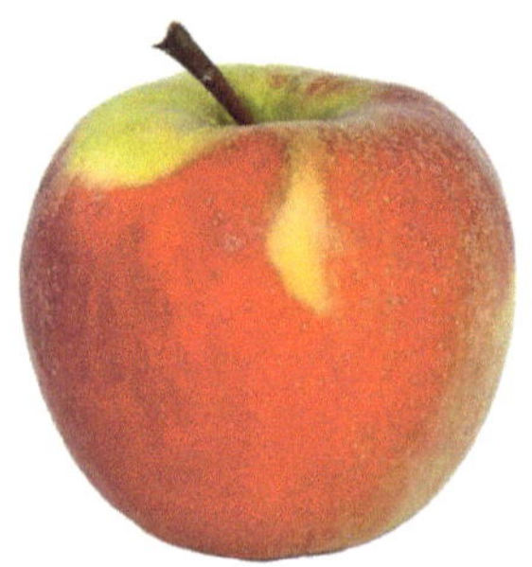

Apples are high in fiber and water

They aid in weight loss, they have antioxidants and they have probiotics.

Here is a list of some healing fruits:

Cherries: Cherries are full of **antioxidants** and **anti-inflammatory** compounds

Strawberries: Rich in vitamin C and provide a good dose of fiber, **folic acid**, manganese and **potassium**

Bananas: Contain high amount of Rutin. Rutin also possesses **antioxidant**, **anti**-inflammatory and **anti-cancer** properties

Mangos: Research has shown **antioxidant** compounds in mango fruit have been found to protect against colon, breast, leukemia and prostate cancers

Papaya: Rich in antioxidants and fights off inflammation and improves digestion

Dragonfruit: Has anti-aging properties, fights off cancer, boosts immune system and lessens the risk of diabetes

Avocado:Contains 20 vitamins and minerals and is a good fat and can be used for skincare as well.

Blueberries: Packed with nutrients and lowers blood pressure and cholesterol.

Kiwi- Used in Chinese medicine this fruit will strengthen your heart and fight off cancer.

Guava- This tropical fruit is amazing in that it packs a punch in that it offers more than 60 percent more potassium than a banana

Pineapple-Asthma fighting, cancer preventing, inflammation stopping super fruit

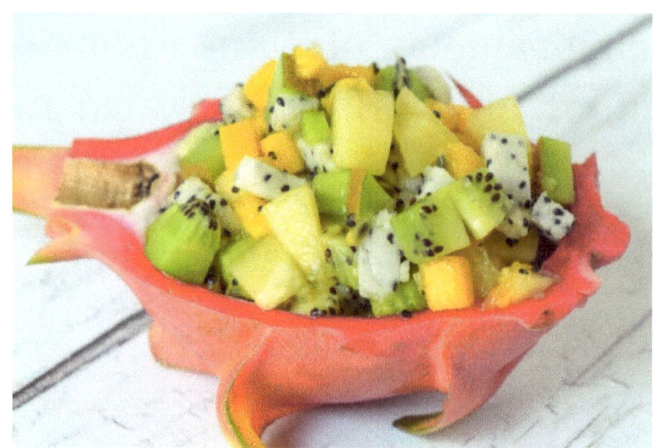

Because almost every single vegetable has healing properties, I won't be breaking them all done. Instead let's focus on the veggies that will deliver the most healing and are delicious as well. My top suggestions are: Brocolli, Cabbage, Spinach, Carrots, celery, cilantro, parsley and mushrooms. This whole combination will make an amazing crockpot dinner in itself!

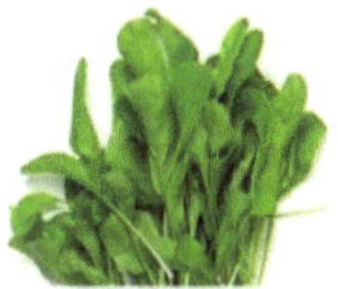

arugula
1 cal/leaf

high in protein, fiber, calcium, iron, magnesium, potassium, and vitamins a, c, k, b6

eat it in salads or in sadwiches and wraps

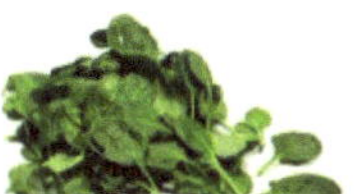

spinach
2 cal/leaf

high in fiber, protein, calcium, iron, magnesium, potassium, and vitamins a, c, e, k, b6

high in sodium

eat it raw in salads, stir-fried, or cooked

mushrooms
2 cal/mushroom

high in fiber, protein, iron, potassium, and vitamins d and b6

eat them stir-fried, sauteed, or roasted

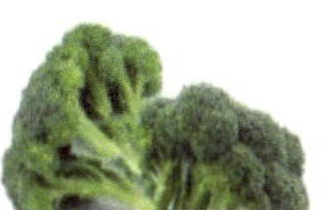

broccoli
3 cal/floret

high in protein, calcium, iron, magnesium, potassium, and vitamins a, c, b6

eat it steamed, roasted, and in salads

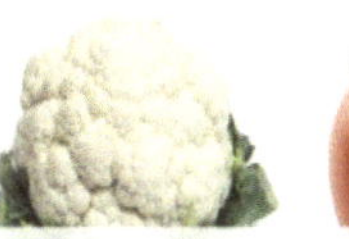

cauliflower
3 cal/floret

high in protein, magnesium, fiber, potassium, and vitamins c, k, b6

high in sugars

eat it steamed, roasted, or in salads

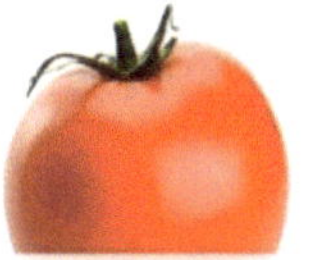

tomatoes
22 cal/tomato

high in magnesium, fiber, potassium, and vitamins a, c, k

high in sugars

eat them raw, in salads, or in sandwiches

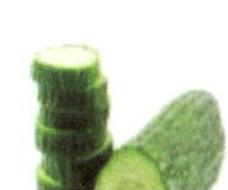

cucumbers
24 cal/cucumber

high in magnesium, potassium, and vitamins a, c, k

high in sugars

eat it raw or in salads

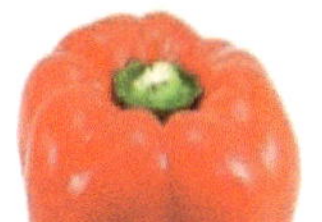

red bell pepper
30 cal/pepper

high in fiber, potassium, and vitamins a, c, k, e, b6

high in sugars

eat it raw, in salads, roasted, or stir-fried

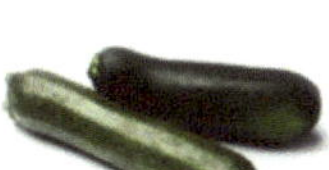

zucchini
31 cal/zucchini

high in fiber, protein, iron, magnesium, potassium, and vitamins a, c, b6

eat it roasted, sauteed, stir fried, or in salads

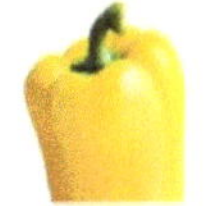

yellow pepper
40 cal/pepper

high in fiber, magnesium, potassium, and vitamins a, c, b6

high in sugars

eat them raw, stir-fried, in salads, or roasted

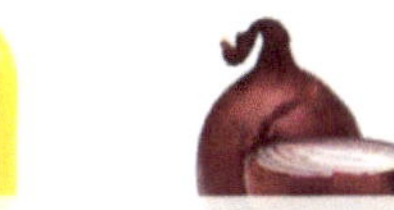

red onions
44 cal/onion

high in fiber, potassium, and vitamins c and b6

high in sugars

eat it roasted, sauteed, stir-fried, or in salads

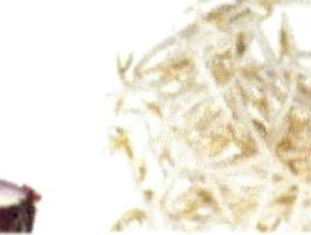

bean sprouts
54 cal/12 oz

high in fiber

high in sugars

eat them in sanwiches, in salads, or stir-fried

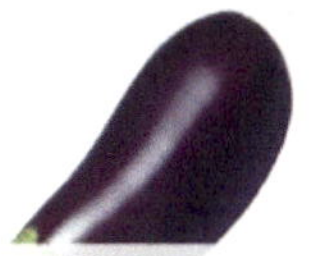

eggplant
110 cal/eggplant

high in magnesium, fiber, potassium, and vitamins c, k, b6

high in sugars

eat them roasted, in salads, or stir-fried

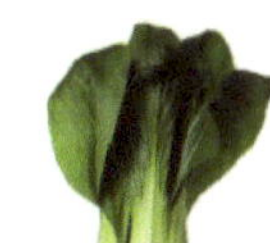

bok choy
2 cal/leaf

high in fiber, protein, iron, calcium, and vitamins a and c

eat it in soups, in salads, or stir-fried

Chapter 2- Fruit Smoothie Recipes

For most of these recipes you will be making blended frozen smoothies. The reason for this is you not only want the texture to be creamy and fulfilling but the ice gives more water content which helps with the weight loss process. The ingredients will be different but the process will be the same for all smoothies. Don't be afraid to add extra ingredients and modify the amounts to your liking.

<u>Instructions:</u>   You will place the cubes of ice in the blender first

Next throw in all of the fruit ingredients.

Follow this with 1 cup of Aloe Vera juice, 2 cups of desired juice recommended for type of smoothie, and 1 cup of water.

First press the crush ice button for 1 minute

Next press the smoothie button on your blender and let it blend until all of the ingredients are perfectly blended. It should look smooth and creamy. Depending on the style of smoothie you want, here are some tips. If you want a more liquified smoothie instead of a creamy one add more juice or water. If you want a creamier smoothie add more ice and 1 banana.

<u>Cherry Passion Smoothie:</u>

1. 5-7 cubes of ice
2. Handful of cherries (5-7 pieces, remove seeds)
3. 5 strawberries
4. 1 Guava
5. 1 Cup Aloe Vera Juice
6. 3-4 Cups Cranberry juice.
7. (Optional) 1 Banana to create creamy texture

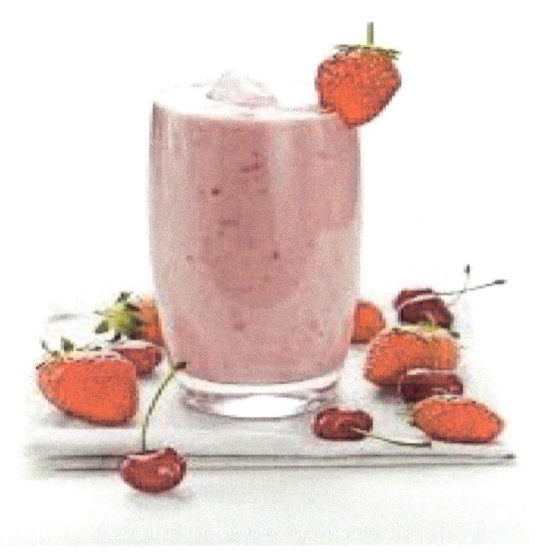

This will make 2 -8oz smoothie drinks

Blueberry Pitaya Crush Smoothie:

Ingredients:

1. 5-7 Cubes of ice

2. Handful of blueberries (6-9 pieces)

3. 1- Dragonfruit

4. 5-8 Chunks of Pinapple

5. 3-4 Cups Apple Juice

6. 1 Cup of Aloe Vera juice or water.

7 (Optional) 1 Banana to create creamy texture

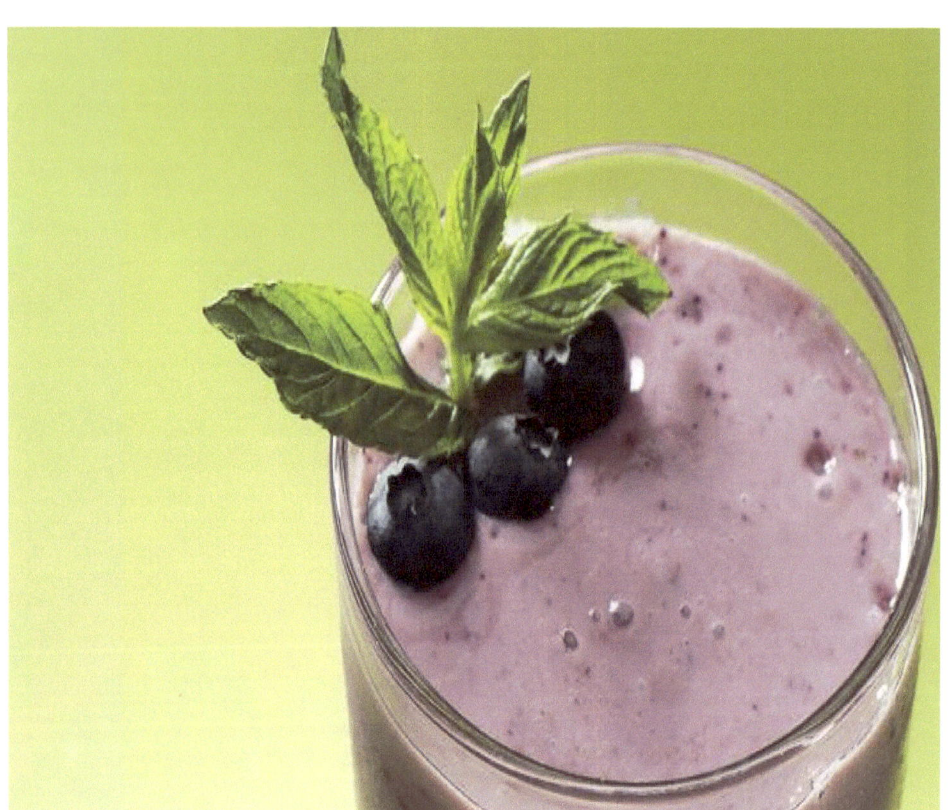

Pinapple Guava Smoothie:

Ingredients:

1.5-7 Cubes of ice

2. Chunks of pinapple (5-7)

3. 5- pieces of rasberries

4. 1 Guava

5. 1 Cup Aloe Vera Juice

6. 3-4 Cups pineapple orange juice.

7.(Optional) 1 Banana to create creamy texture

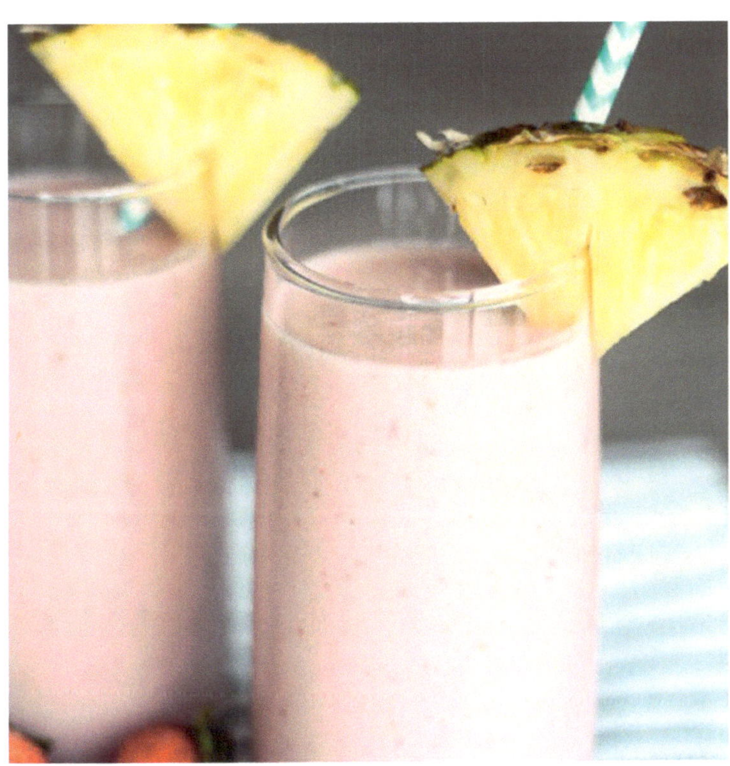

Papaya Peach Smoothie:

Ingredients:

1.5-7 Cubes of ice

2.Handful of Peaches (6-8 pieces)

3. 1 Papaya(Remove seeds, cut in chunks)
4. 2-4 Strawberries
5. 3-4 Cups Peach Cranberry Juice.

6.(Optional) 1 Banana to create creamy texture

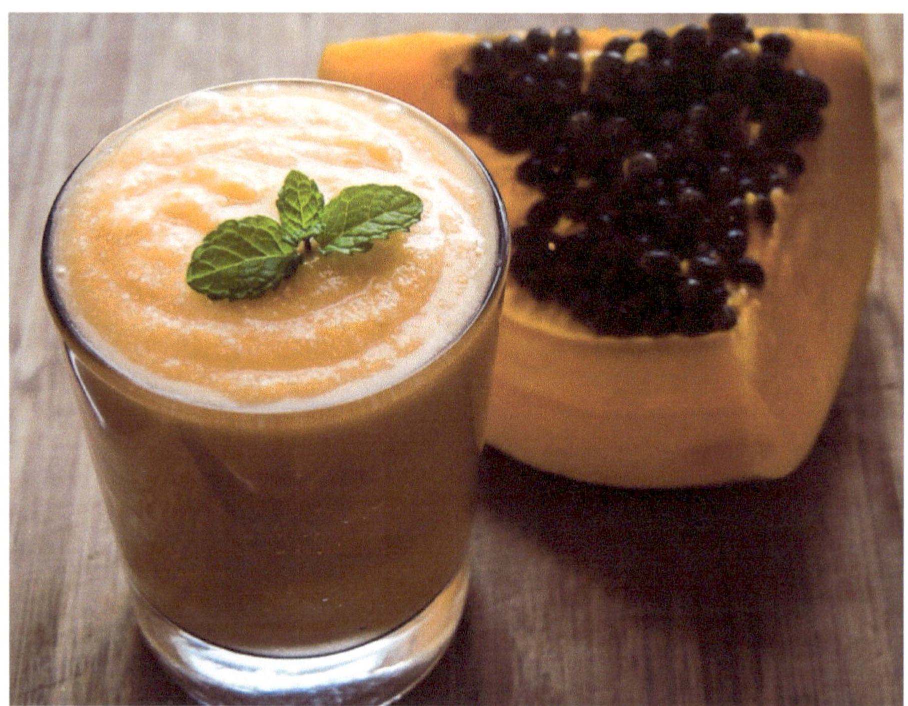

Ginger Mango Madness Smoothie:

<u>Ingredients:</u>

1. 5-7 Cubes of ice
2. Handful of peaches (5-7 pieces)
3. 2- Mangos-Cut into chunks
4. 1 Cup of shaved Ginger or Ginger powder
5. 1- Lime
6. 3-4 Cups Mango juice.

7.(Optional) 1 Banana to create creamy texture

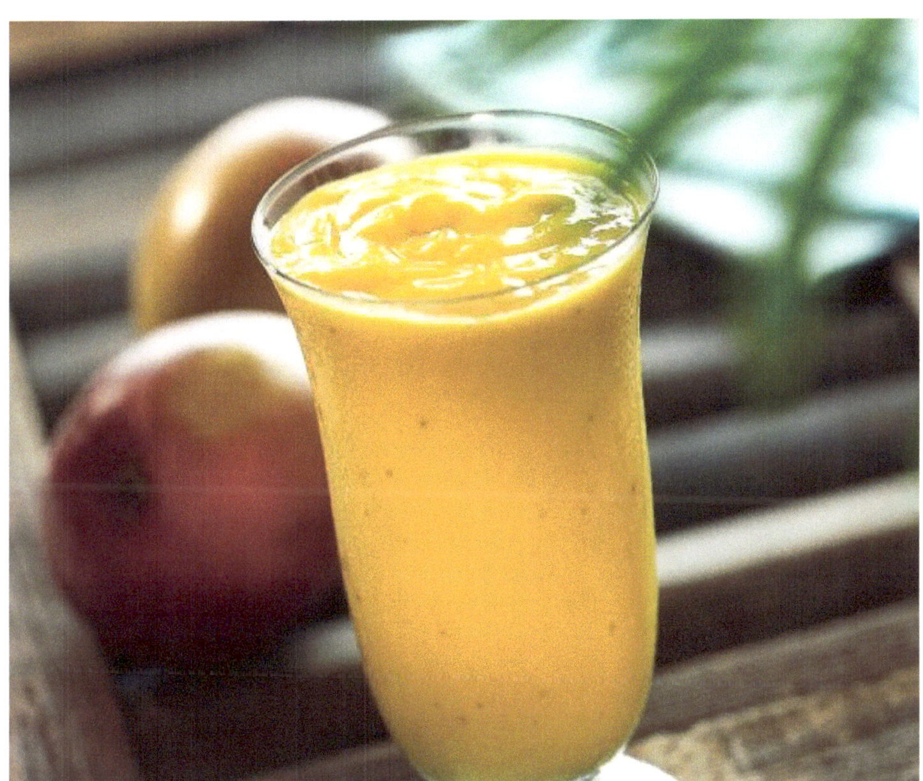

<u>Watermelon Ginger Spice Smoothie:</u>

<u>Ingredients:</u>

1. 5-7 Cubes of ice

2. Handful of watermelon (10 pieces)

3. 1 Cup of Ginger Powder or Shaved Ginger

4. 1 Piece Jalapeno (Cut into small pieces)

5. 1- Lemon

6. 3-4 Cups Aloe Vera Watermelon Juice.

7.(Optional) 1 Banana to create creamy texture

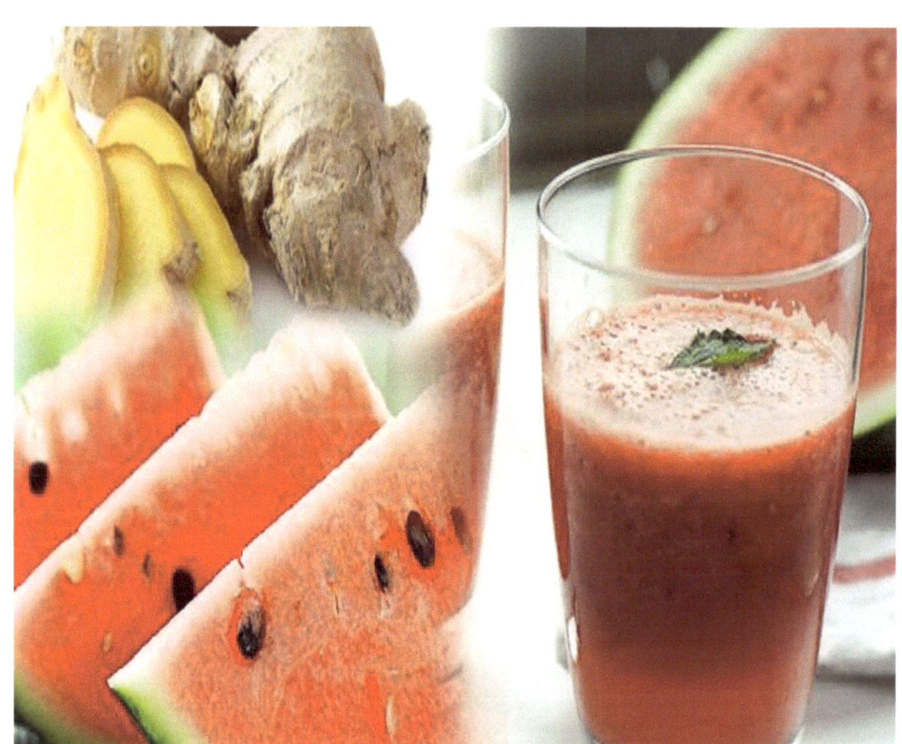

Tropical Explosion Smoothie:

Ingredients:

1. 5-7 Cubes of ice

2. Handful of peaches (5-7 pieces)
3. Handful of rasberries (5-7 pieces)
4. Handful of blueberries(4-6 pieces)
5. Handful of kiwi (4 whole pieces)
6. 1- Guava

7. 3-4 Cups Pineapple Mango juice.

8.(Optional) 1 Banana to create creamy texture

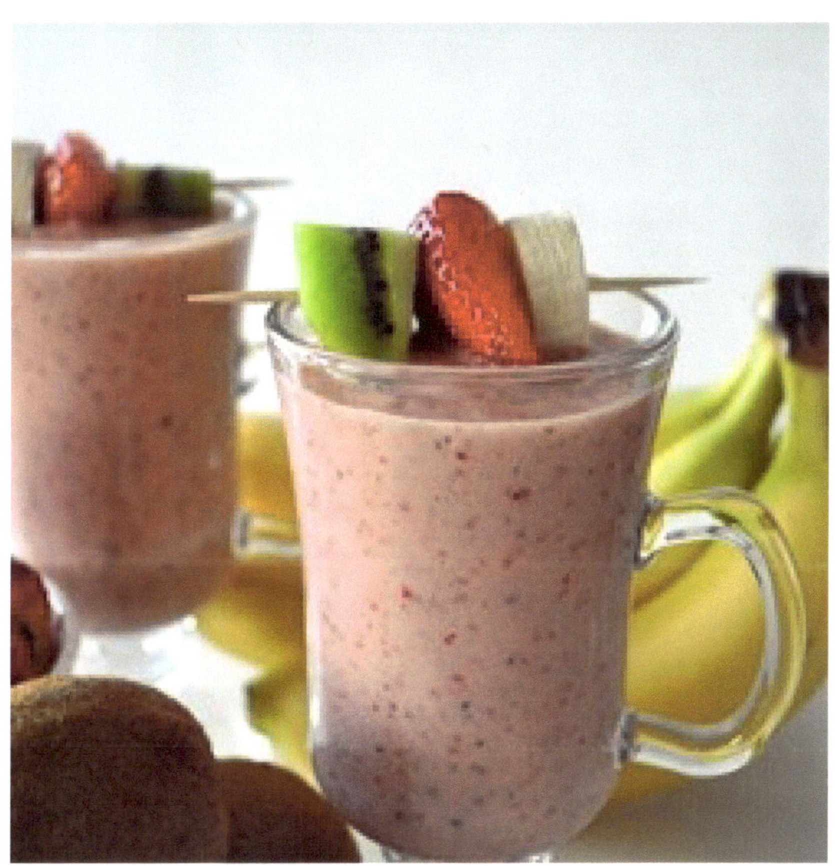

Dragonfruit Berry Smoothie:

Ingredients:

1. 5-7 Cubes of ice

2. Handful of rasberries (5-7 pieces)

3. Handful of blueberries(4-6 pieces)

4. Handful of strawberries(5 pieces)

5. 1- Cup of Coconut Water

6. 3-4 Cups Cranberry Apple juice.

7.(Optional) 1 Banana to create creamy texture

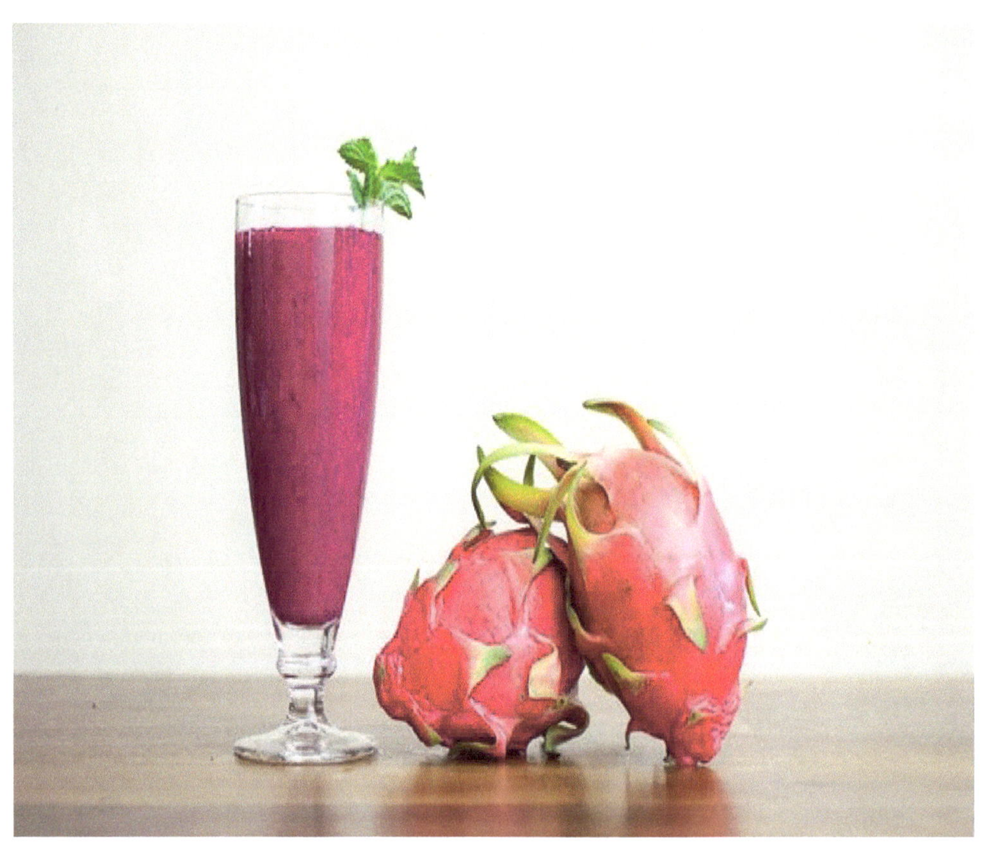

Chapter 3- Veggie Smoothie Recipes

In any of the smoothies you can add vegetables in order to complete the meal. Depending on the taste and desired result of your smoothie certain combinations can help with weight loss and to aid with health issues. The following vegetables have strong healing properties and are tasty in any smoothie.

Spinach:

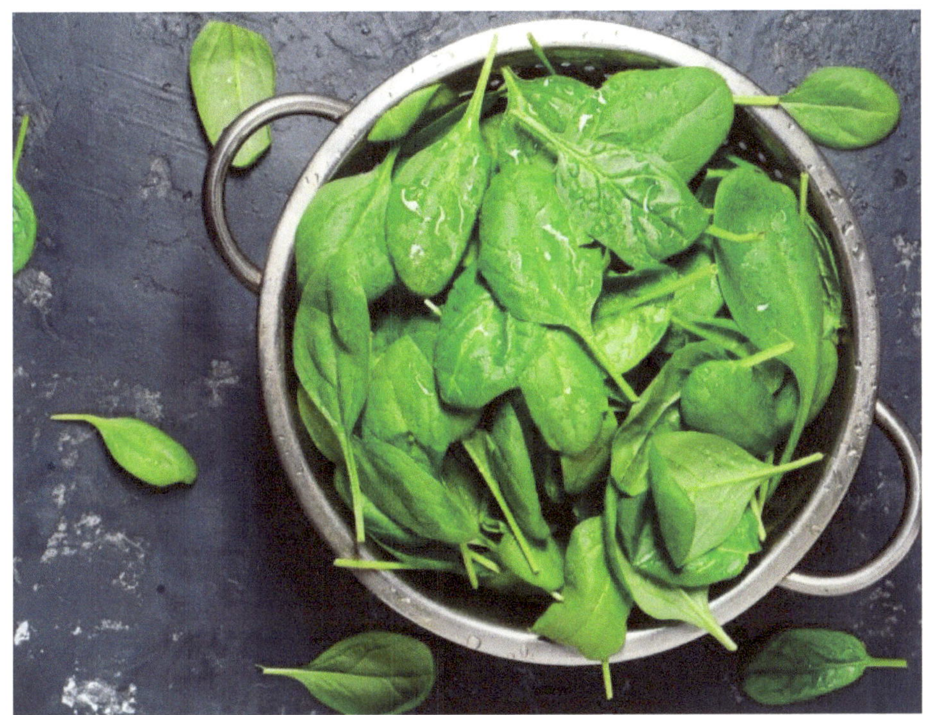

If you don't already know this spinach is a super food. Popeye was trying to tell you! It makes you stronger and can help you fight off diseases. Consuming spinach regularly can help with improving blood glucose control in people with <u>diabetes</u>, lowering the risk of <u>cancer</u>, and improving bone health, as well as supplying minerals and <u>vitamins</u>.

Cilantro:

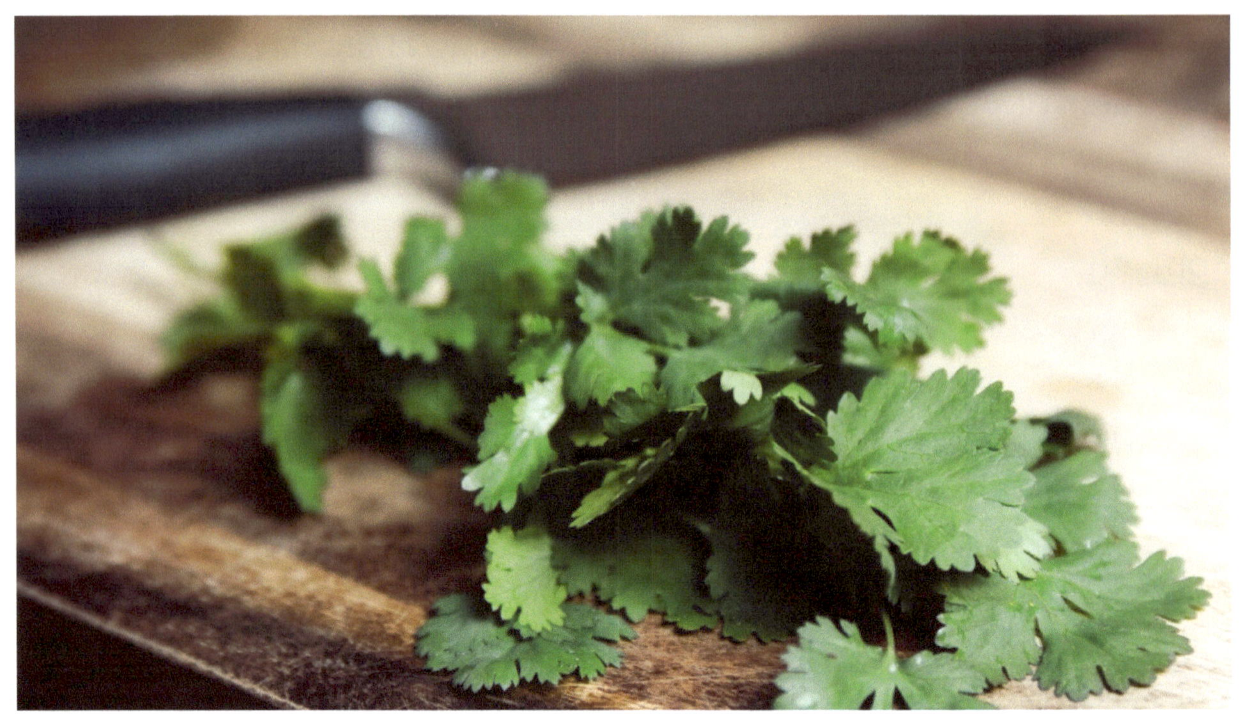

<u>Cilantro </u>is a Mediterranean herb that not only smells good but adds flavor to any meal! Some of the benefits for eating this daily are:

Lowers cholesterol and blood pressure

Has plenty of Vitamin A,C,E,K, Calcium and magnesium

Helps build strong bones, teeth and hair

Celery:

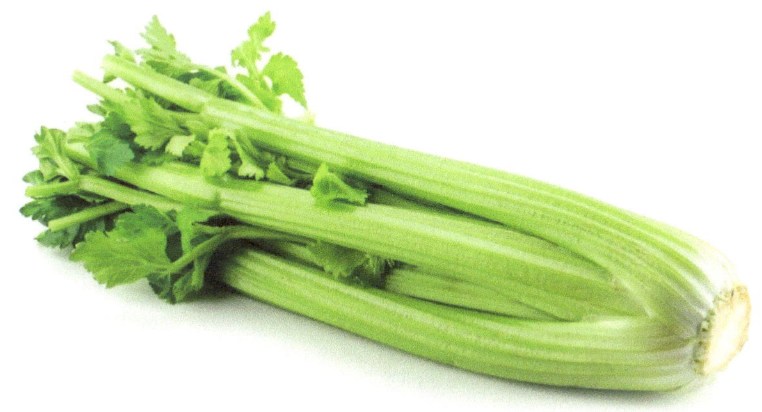

Celery is a heavely water based vegetable but it has a lot of cancer fighting properties. A great juice to drink is a combination of celery, cucumber and lime. The combination of those will help make your heart stronger and fight off inflammation. This is a wonderful and powerful recipe for people with Chron's disease.

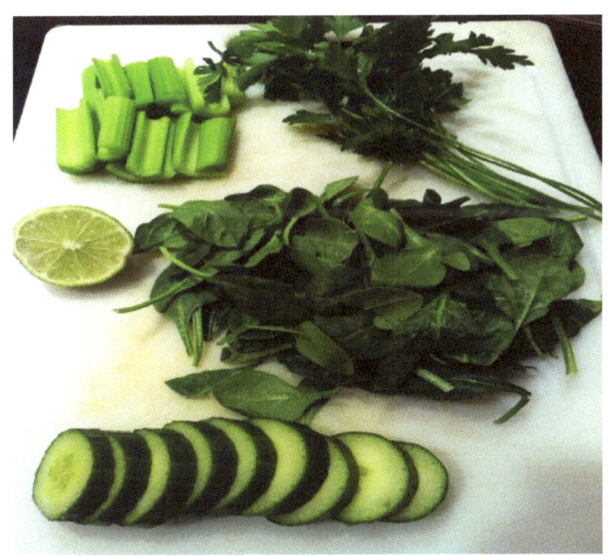

Ginger:

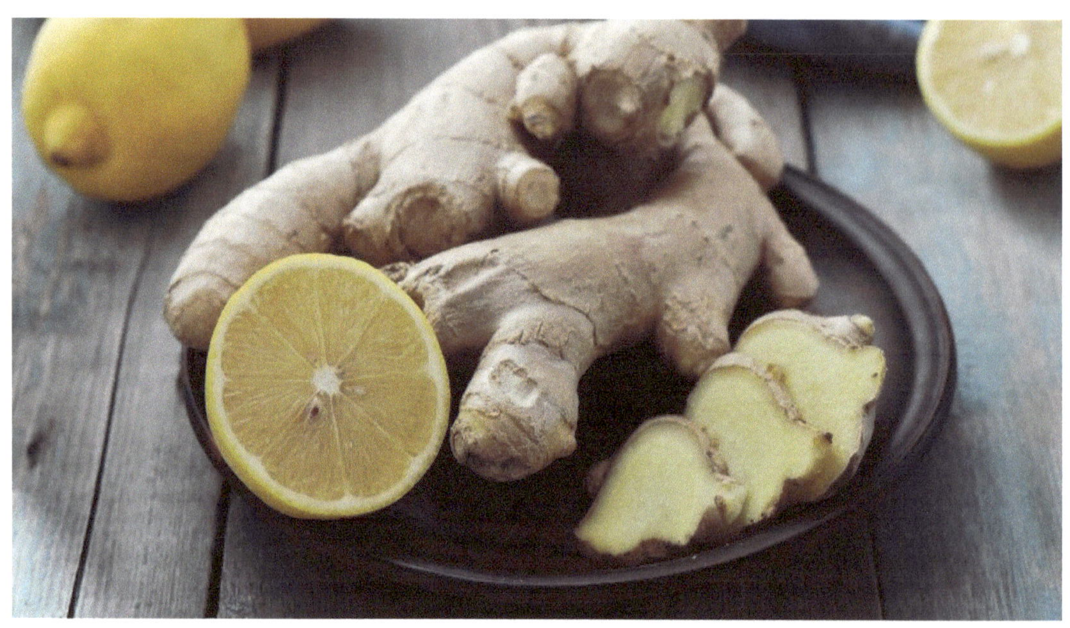

   Ginger is my all time favorite secret ingredient for everything! It helps soothe all stomach ailments. Combine it with cinnamon and you will feel amazing. It helps regulate you and has strong healing properties as well. Ginger is perfect for new moms. It helps control morning sickness and nausea. It fights inflammation and helps aid against osteoporosis. Plus, it is extremely tasty. Ginger teas are also a great way to calm your nerves and help you sleep better. Combine milk, ginger, cinnamon and lemon to make the tea.

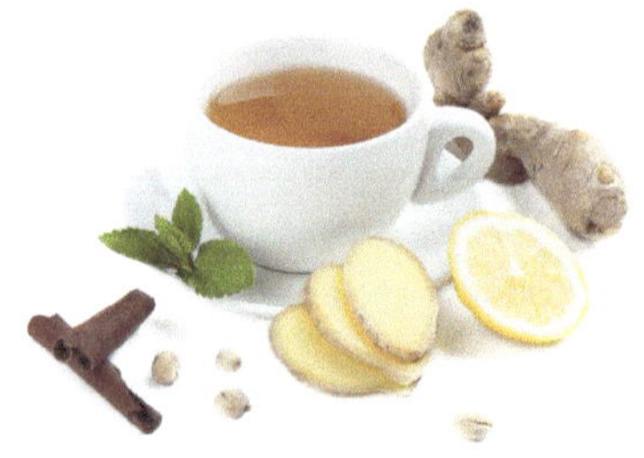

Chia Seeds:

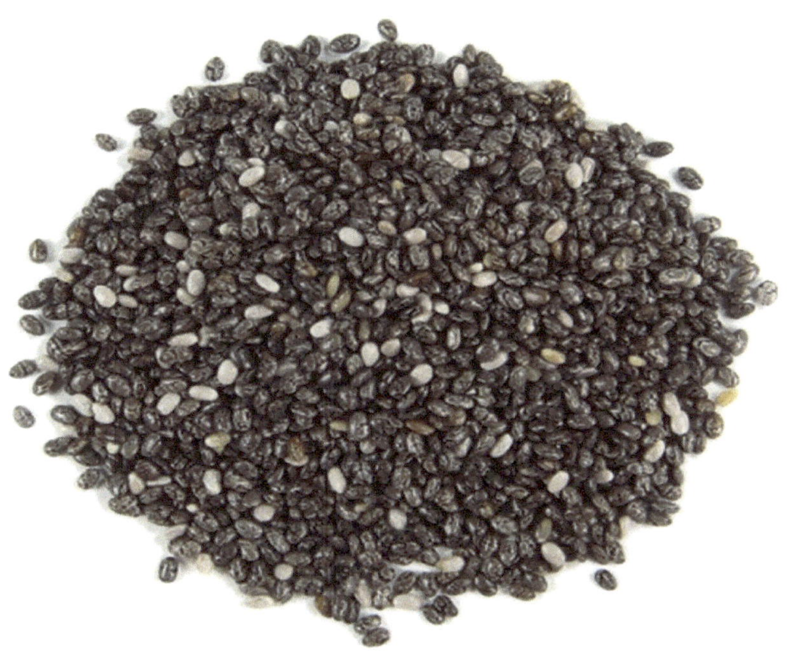

These tiny magical seeds are amazing! They pack so much nutrients and they don't get enough credit for all of the health benefits they give. They are an excellent source of **omega**-3 fatty acids, rich in **antioxidants,** and they provide **fiber, iron, and calcium. Omega**-3 fatty acids help raise HDL **cholesterol,** the "good" **cholesterol** that protects against **heart** attack and **stroke.** **You have to put these on everything you eat and drink.** They don't even taste like anything. Therefore, one scoop of these on anything is really easy to do. Try it out for 1 week and then notice how your body adjusts and feels.

<u>**Chia Peachy Pear Smoothie:**</u>

<u>Ingredients:</u>

1. 5-7 Cubes of ice
2. Handful of peaches (5-7 pieces)
3. Handful of pears(4-6 pieces)
4. 1 Cup of Chia seeds
5. 1- Cup of Coconut Water
6. 3-4 Cups Apple Mango juice.

7.(Optional) 1 Banana to create creamy texture

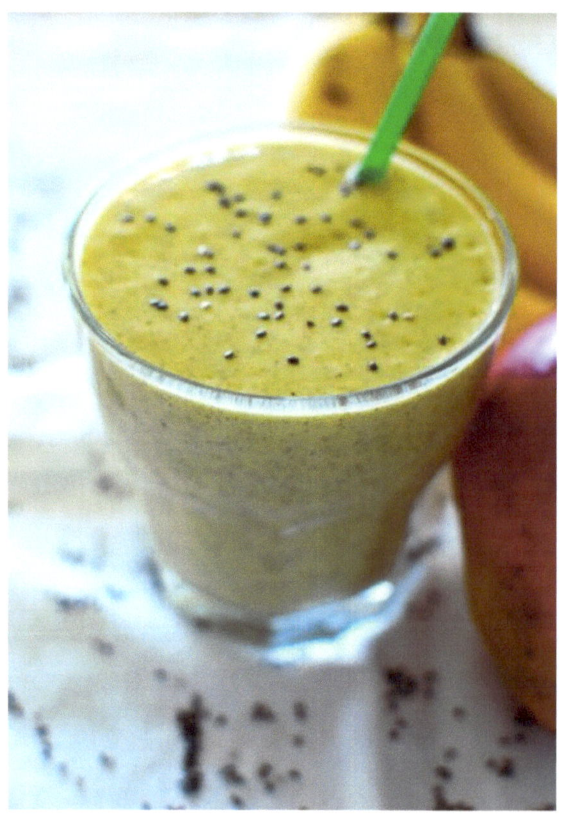

<u>**Green Apple Tummy Smash Smoothie:**</u>

<u>Ingredients:</u>

1. 5-7 Cubes of ice
2. Handful of apples (5-7 pieces)
3. Handful of pears (4-6 pieces)
4. Handful of spinach(1 cup)
5. 1- Cucumber sliced
6. 1- Cup of Coconut water
7. 3-4 Cups Apple juice.

8.(Optional) 1 Banana to create creamy texture

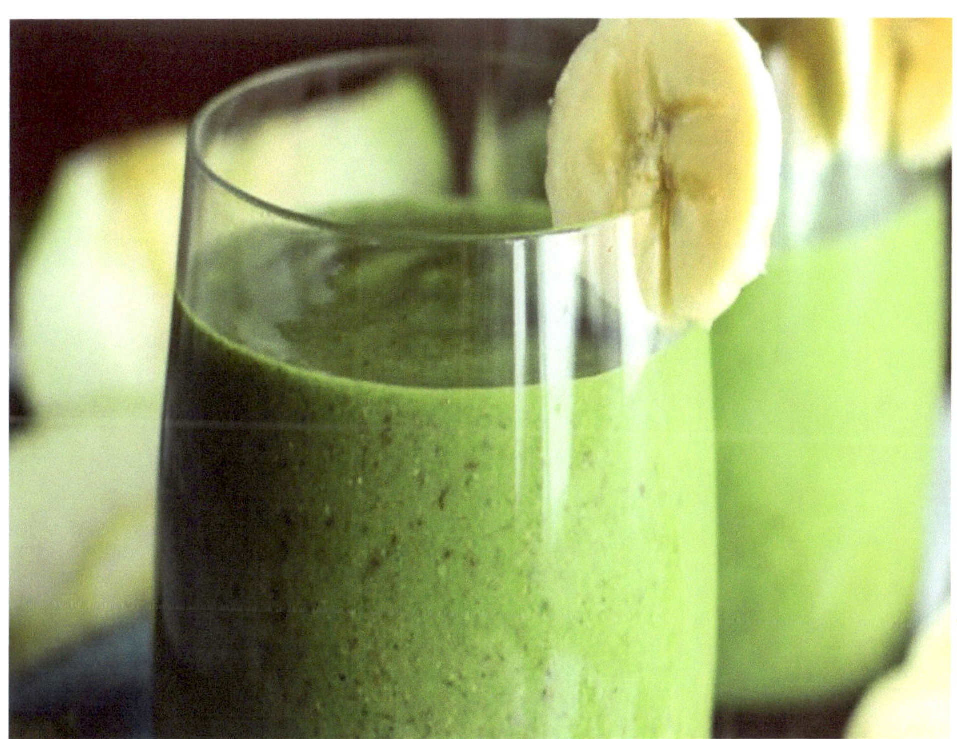

<u>Green Lean Energy Boost Smoothie:</u>

<u>Ingredients:</u>

1. 5-7 Cubes of ice
2. A bushel of cilantro or parsley
3. A cup of spinach or kale
4. 1- Lemon
5. 1- Tablespoon of powder or shaved ginger
6. 1- Cup of Coconut Water
7. 3-4 Cups of Aloe Very juice.

8.(Optional) 1 Banana to create creamy texture

9.(Optional) Sprinkle chia seeds on top

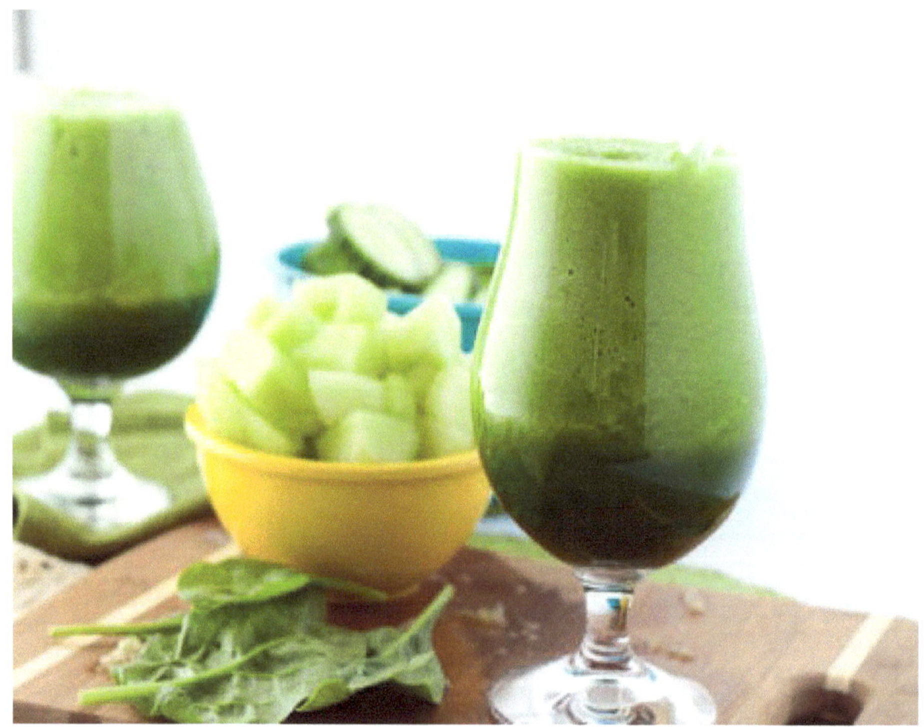

<u>Cinnamon Sleepytime Smoothie:</u>

<u>Ingredients:</u>

1. 5-7 Cubes of ice
2. 1- Cup of Ginger powder or shaved
3. 1- Cup of Cinnamon
4. 1- Teaspoon Turmeric
5. 1/2- Cup of Spinach
6. 2- Cups of Almond Milk
7. 1- Cup of Water.

8.(Optional) 1 Banana to create creamy texture

9. (Optional) 1 Cup of Almonds

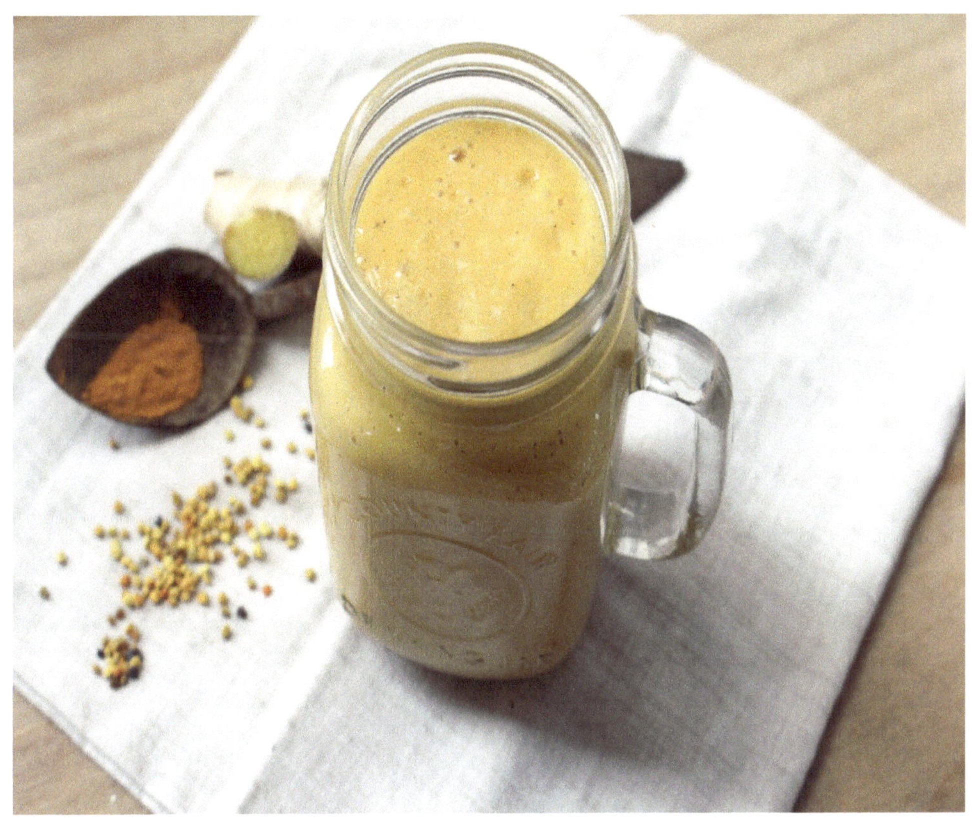

Lemon Power Zing Smoothie:

<u>Ingredients:</u>

1. 5-7 Cubes of ice
2. 1- Lemon
3. 1- Cup of Ginger powder or shaved
4. 1- Guava
5. 1/2- Cup of cilantro
6. 1- Cup of Coconut or AloeVera Water
7. 3-4 Cups Pineapple juice.

7.(Optional) 1 Banana to create creamy texture

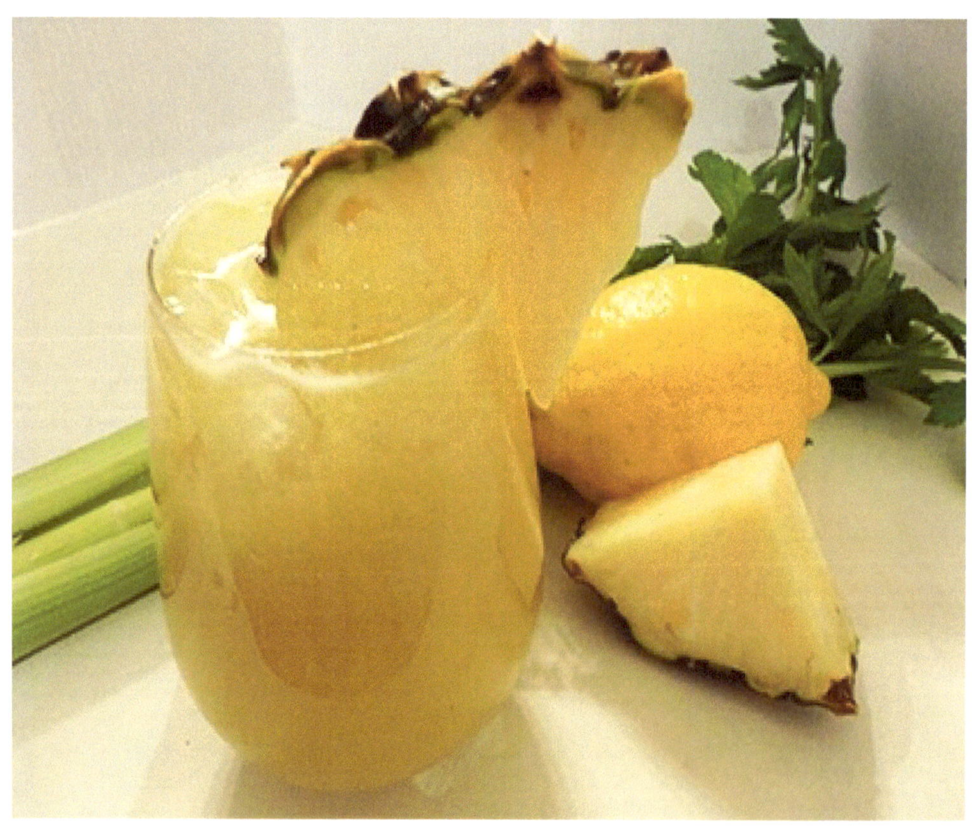

Fruits and vegetables are not only good snacks throughout the day, but they make for wonderful lunch and dinner meals as well. You will never hear of anyone overdosing on fruit or someone getting obese off a fruit diet. That's because food is medicine and fruits and vegetables are really all your body needs. Now, I do understand for certain health conditions you are required to eat specific things that may include meat for some people or omission of certain fruit sugars for others. However, you can use the fruit and veggie diet as a preventative measure. Start changing your eating habits now and your future self will have a higher chance to fight off diseases and you will live longer!

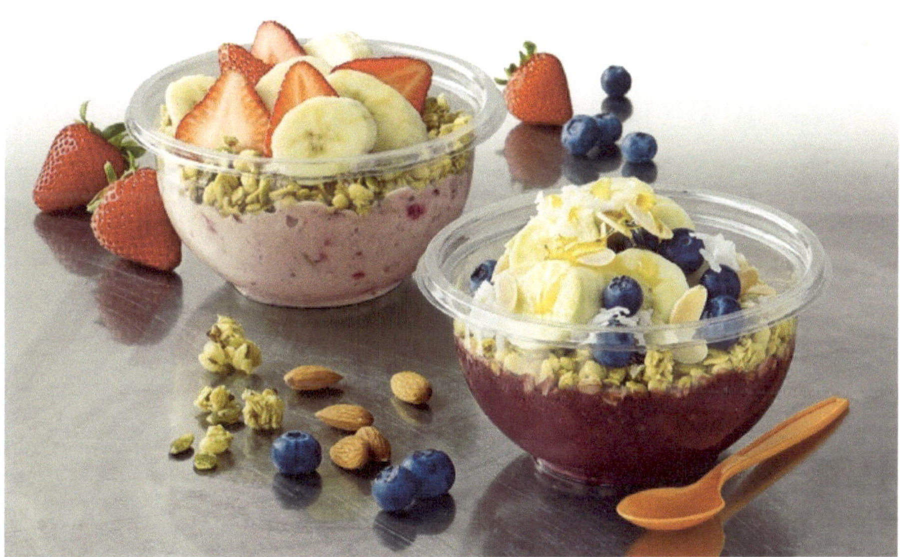

Honey Pitaya Fruit Bowl:

<u>Ingredients:</u>

1. 5-7 Cubes of ice
2. 1- Dragonfruit
3. 2- Whole bananas sliced
4. Handful of rasberries (5-7 pieces)
5. Handful of blueberries(5-7 pieces)
6. Handful of strawberries(5 pieces)
7. 1- Cup of granola or oats
8. 1- Cup of coconut chips
9. Drizzle of Honey

Instructions:

1.Blend the ice and handful of blueberries with the dragonfruit

2. Pour this in a bowl

3. Add all of the other ingredients of fruit first

4. Add then granola and coconut chips on top

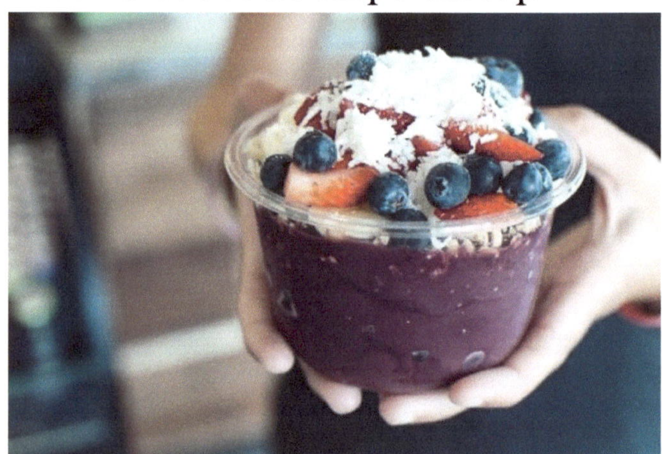

5. Drizzle honey

This meal is very filling and satisfying!

Mango Tango Fruit Bowl

1. 1-2 Cups of Greek yogurt peach flavor
2. 1-2 Mangos
3. 2- Whole bananas sliced
4. Handful of peaches (5-7 pieces)
5. Handful of apricots(5-7 pieces)
6. Handful of rasberries(5 pieces)
7. 1- Cup of granola or oats
8. 1- Cup of Chia seeds
9. Drizzle of Honey

Instructions:

1. Place the yogurt in the bowl first.
2. Add all of the sliced fruits
3. Add the granola
4. Top off with the Chia seeds and drizzle of honey.

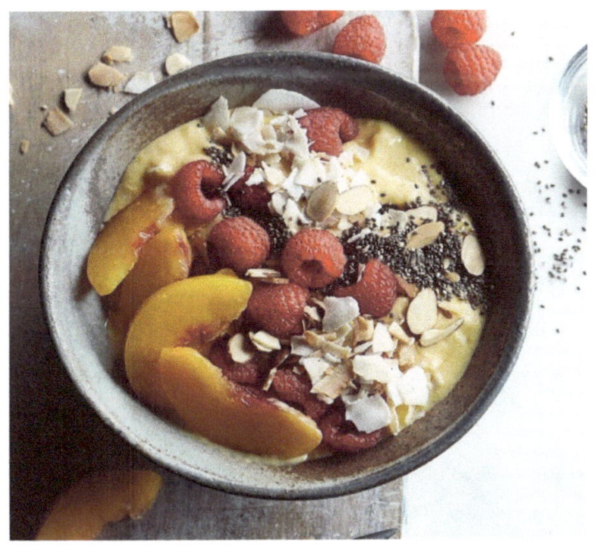

Fruit Salad Bowl:

<u>Ingredients:</u>

1. Package of Mixed Leafy Greens(Spinach,Lettuce,Kale)
2. 1-2 Apples
3. 1-2 Pears
4. 1 Cucumber
5. 1 Tomato
6. 1 Avocado
7. Handful of rasberries (5-7 pieces)
8. Handful of blueberries(5-7 pieces)
9. Handful of strawberries(5 pieces)
10.1- Cup of black olives
11.1 Cup of Chia Seeds
12. Dressing (Lemon,Apple ciderVinagrette)

Instructions:
1.Cut up all of the fruit into small chunks
2. Pour the leafy greens in a bowl
3. Create the dressing. Simple add Apple cider vinegar, lemon juice and a pinch of oil into a bowl
4. Mix the leafy greens with the dressing.
5. Add all of the fruit and avocado

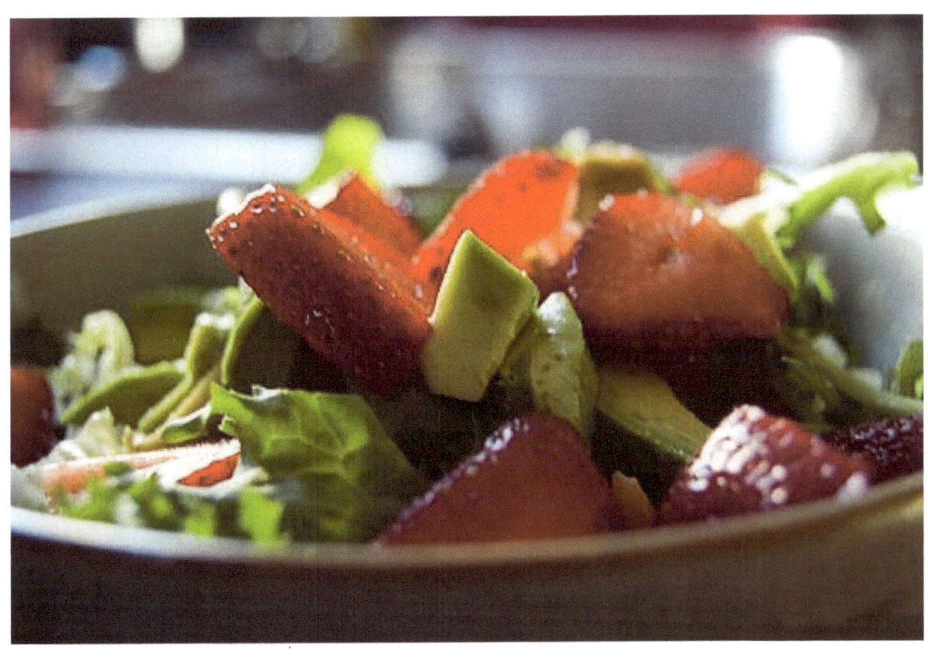

If you stuck to this new meal plan then Congratulations. Having will power and discipline is half the battle. All of the smoothie recipes on here are extremely powerful, delicious and can be used in any combination you see fit. When it comes to eating healthy as long as you treat your body good with foods packed with vitamins and nutrients you will start to see results. You will feel more energized. You will start to think a lot clearer. You will look at the world with a new appreciation and you will see physical results as well. You have to start with your insides before you will reap the rewards on the outside.

Don't be afraid to add different fruits and vegetables to each recipe. Once you find a winning combination for yourself-stick to it! In the beginning of the book I described that you want to use these recipes as a substitute for meals until you get on a routine of changing your eating habits. After you have reached your goal, your new normal would be to incorporate one or 2 of these smoothies as your daily meal or as a pick me up in between snacks. You will start to save money as well. When you prepare more foods at home and eat fruits and vegetables you will spend less on your groceries. This is an all-around win-win. Take this smoothie diet challenge and I promise you will feel like a million bucks!

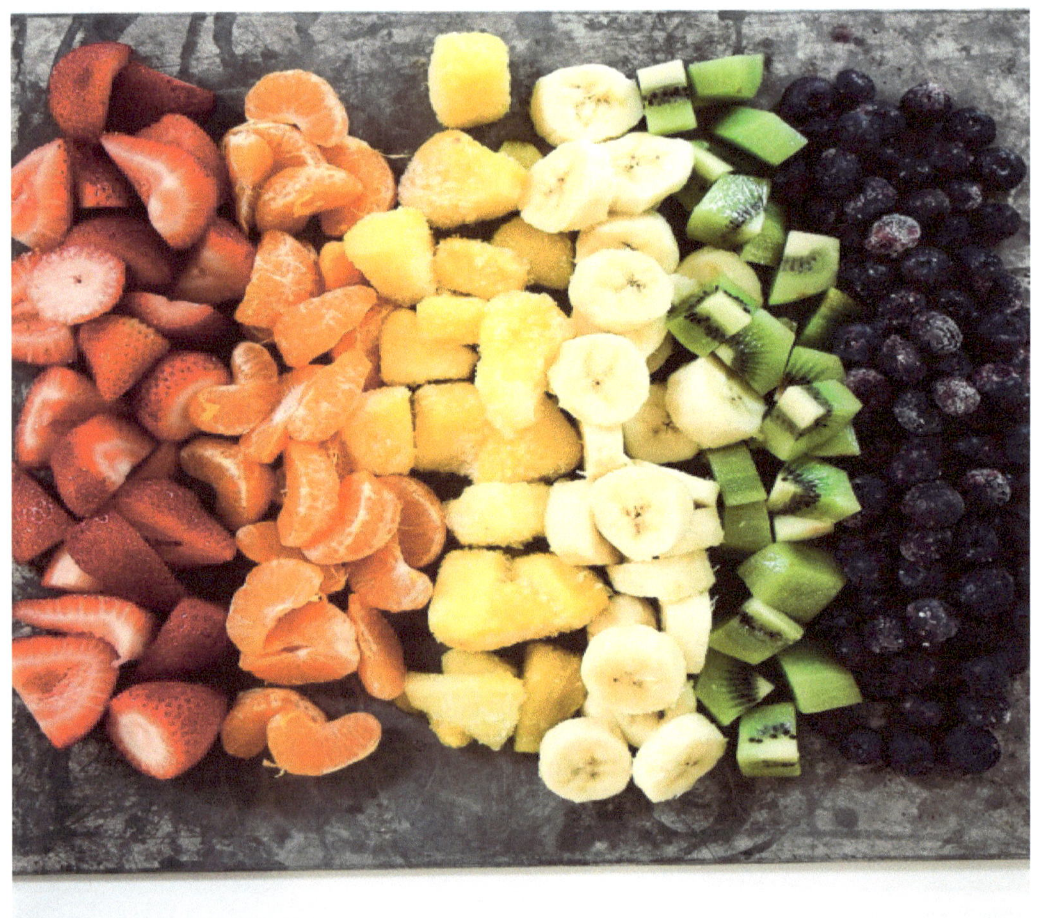